Best Plant Based Diet Cookbook

Best Cookbook with Practical Plant Based Diet Recipes for Eat Healthy Foods, The Best Easy Way for Lose Weight

Tamy Carola

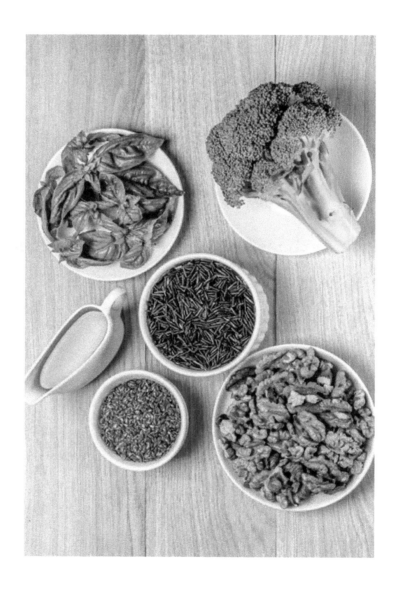

Table of Contents

Introduction

A plant-based diet is a diet based primarily on whole plant foods. It is identical to the regular diet we're used to already, except that it leaves out foods that are not exclusively from plants. Hence, a plant-based diet does away with all types of animal-sourced foods, hydrogenated oils, refined sugars, and processed foods. A whole food plant-based diet comprises not just fruits and vegetables; it also consists of unprocessed or barely-processed oils with healthy monounsaturated fats (like extra-virgin olive oil), whole grains, legumes (essentially lentils and beans), seeds and nuts, as well as herbs and spices. What makes a plant-based meal (or any meal) fun is the manner with which you make them; the seasoning process; and the combination process that contributes to a fantastic flavor and makes every meal unique and enjoyable. There are lots of delicious recipes (all plant-centered), which will prove helpful in when you intend making mouthwatering, healthy plant-based dishes for personal or household consumption. Provided you're eating these plant-based foods regularly, you'll have very problems with fat or diseases that result from bad dietary habits, and there would be no need for excessive calorie tracking. Plant-based diet recipes are versatile; they range from colorful Salads to Lentil Stews, and Bean Burritos. The recipes also draw influences from around the globe, with Mexican, Chinese, European, Indian cuisines all part of the vast array of plant-based recipes available to choose from. Why You Ought to Reduce Your Intake of Processed and Animal-Based Foods. You have likely heard over and over that processed food has adverse effects on your health. You might have also been told repeatedly to stay away from foods with lots of preservatives; nevertheless, nobody ever offered any genuine or concrete facts about why you ought to avoid these foods and why they are unsafe. Consequently, let us properly dissect it to help you properly comprehend why you ought to stay away from these healthy eating offenders. They have massive habit-forming characteristics. Humans have a predisposition towards being addicted to some specific foods; however, the reality is that the fault is not wholly ours. Every one of the unhealthy treats we relish now and then triggers the dopamine release in our brains. This creates a pleasurable effect in our brain, but the excitement is usually short-lived. The discharged dopamine additionally causes an attachment connection gradually, and this is the reason some people consistently go back to eat certain unhealthy foods even when they know it's unhealthy and unnecessary. You can get rid of this by taking out that inducement completely. They are sugar-laden and plenteous in glucose-fructose syrup. Animal-based and processed foods are laden with refined sugars and glucose-fructose syrup which has almost no beneficial food nutrient. An ever-increasing number of studies are affirming what several people presumed from the start; that genetically modified foods bring about inflammatory bowel disease, which consequently makes it increasingly difficult for the body to assimilate essential nutrients. The disadvantages that result from your body being unable to assimilate essential nutrients from consumed foods rightly cannot be overemphasized. Processed and animal-based food products contain plenteous amounts of refined carbohydrates. Indeed, your body requires carbohydrates to give it the needed energy to run body capacities. In any case, refining carbs dispenses with the fundamental supplements; in the way that refining entire grains disposes of the whole grain part. What remains, in the wake of refining, is what's considered as empty carbs or empty calories. These can negatively affect the metabolic system in your body by sharply increasing your blood sugar and insulin quantities. They contain lots of synthetic ingredients. At the point when your body is taking in non-natural ingredients, it regards them as foreign substances. Your body treats them as a health threat. Your body isn't accustomed to identifying synthetic compounds like sucralose or these synthesized sugars. Hence, in defense of your health against this foreign "aggressor," your body does what it's capable of to safeguard your health. It sets off an immune reaction to tackle this "enemy" compound, which indirectly weakens your body's general disease alertness, making you susceptible to illnesses. The concentration and energy expended by your body in ensuring your immune system remain safe could instead be devoted somewhere else. They contain constituent elements that set off an excitable reward sensation in your body. A part of processed and animal-based foods contain compounds like glucose-fructose syrup, monosodium glutamate, and specific food dyes that can trigger some addiction. They rouse your body to receive a benefit in return whenever you consume them. Monosodium glutamate, for example, is added to many store-bought baked foods. This additive slowly conditions your palates to relish the taste. It gets mental just by how your brain interrelates with your taste sensors.

This reward-centric arrangement makes you crave it increasingly, which ends up exposing you to the danger of over consuming calories.

For animal protein, usually, the expression "subpar" is used to allude to plant proteins since they generally have lower levels of essential amino acids as against animal-sourced protein. Nevertheless, what the vast majority don't know is that large amounts of essential amino acids can prove detrimental to your health. Let me break it down further for you.

Chocolate Avocado Ice Cream

Preparation Time: 1 hour and 10 minutes

Cooking Time: 0 minute

Servings: 2

Ingredients:

    4.5 ounces avocado, peeled, pitted

    1/2 cup cocoa powder, unsweetened

    1 tablespoon vanilla extract, unsweetened

    1/2 cup and 2 tablespoons maple syrup

    13.5 ounces coconut milk, unsweetened

    1/2 cup water

Directions:

1. Add avocado in a food processor along with milk and then pulse for 2 minutes until smooth.
2. Add remaining ingredients, blend until mixed, and then tip the pudding in a freezer-proof container.
3. Place the container in a freezer and chill for freeze for 4 hours until firm, whisking every 20 minutes after 1 hour.
4. Serve straight away.

Nutrition:

      Calories: 80.7 Cal

      Fat: 7.1 g

      Carbs: 6 g

      Protein: 0.6 g

      Fiber: 2 g

Watermelon Mint Popsicles

Preparation Time: 8 hours and 5 minutes

Cooking Time: 0 minute

Servings: 8

Ingredients:

20 mint leaves, diced

6 cups watermelon chunks

3 tablespoons lime juice

Directions:

Add watermelon in a food processor along with lime juice and then pulse for 15 seconds until smooth.

Pass the watermelon mixture through a strainer placed over a bowl, remove the seeds and then stir mint into the collected watermelon mixture.

Take eight Popsicle molds, pour in prepared watermelon mixture, and freeze for 2 hours until slightly firm.

Then insert popsicle sticks and continue freezing for 6 hours until solid.

Serve straight away

Nutrition:

Calories: 90 Cal

Fat: 0 g

Carbs: 23 g

Protein: 0 g

Fiber: 0 g

Mango Coconut Chia Pudding

Preparation Time: 2 hours and 5 minutes

Cooking Time: 0 minute

Servings: 1

Ingredients:

- 1 medium mango, peeled, cubed
- 1/4 cup chia seeds
- 2 tablespoons coconut flakes
- 1 cup coconut milk, unsweetened
- 1 1/2 teaspoons maple syrup

Directions:

Take a bowl, place chia seeds in it, whisk in milk until combined, and then stir in maple syrup.

Cover the bowl with a plastic wrap; it should touch the pudding mixture and refrigerate for 2 hours until the pudding has set.

Then puree mango until smooth, top it evenly over pudding, sprinkle with coconut flakes and serve.

Nutrition:

Calories: 159 Cal

Fat: 9 g

Carbs: 17 g

Protein: 3 g

Fiber: 6 g

Brownie Energy Bites

Preparation Time: 1 hour and 10 minutes

Cooking Time: 0 minute

Servings: 2

Ingredients:

- 1/2 cup walnuts
- 1 cup Medjool dates, chopped
- 1/2 cup almonds
- 1/8 teaspoon salt
- 1/2 cup shredded coconut flakes
- 1/3 cup and 2 teaspoons cocoa powder, unsweetened

Directions:

Place almonds and walnuts in a food processor and pulse for 3 minutes until the dough starts to come together.

Add remaining ingredients, reserving ¼ cup of coconut and pulse for 2 minutes until incorporated.

Shape the mixture into balls, roll them in remaining coconut until coated, and refrigerate for 1 hour.

Serve straight away

Nutrition:

Calories: 174.6 Cal

Fat: 8.1 g

Carbs: 25.5 g

Protein: 4.1 g

Fiber: 4.4 g

Strawberry Coconut Ice Cream

Preparation Time: 5 minutes

Cooking Time: 0 minute

Servings: 4

Ingredients:

>   4 cups frouncesen strawberries
>
>   1 vanilla bean, seeded
>
>   28 ounces coconut cream
>
>   1/2 cup maple syrup

Directions:

>   Place cream in a food processor and pulse for 1 minute until soft peaks come together.
>
>   Then tip the cream in a bowl, add remaining ingredients in the blender and blend until thick mixture comes together.
>
>   Add the mixture into the cream, fold until combined, and then transfer ice cream into a freezer-safe bowl and freeze for 4 hours until firm, whisking every 20 minutes after 1 hour.
>
>   Serve straight away.

Nutrition:

    Calories: 100 Cal

    Fat: 100 g

    Carbs: 100 g

    Protein: 100 g

    Fiber: 100 g

Salted Caramel Chocolate Cups

Preparation Time: 5 minutes

Cooking Time: 2 minutes

Servings: 12

Ingredients:

¼ teaspoon sea salt granules

1 cup dark chocolate chips, unsweetened

2 teaspoons coconut oil

6 tablespoons caramel sauce

Directions:

Take a heatproof bowl, add chocolate chips and oil, stir until mixed, then microwave for 1 minute until melted, stir chocolate and continue heating in the microwave for 30 seconds.

Take twelve mini muffin tins, line them with muffin liners, spoon a little bit of chocolate mixture into the tins, spread the chocolate in the bottom and along the sides, and freeze for 10 minutes until set.

Then fill each cup with ½ tablespoon of caramel
sauce, cover with remaining chocolate and
freeze for another 2salt0 minutes until set.
When ready to eat, peel off liner from the cup,
sprinkle with sauce, and serve.

Nutrition:

Calories: 80 Cal

Fat: 5 g

Carbs: 10 g

Protein: 1 g

Fiber: 0.5 g

Chocolate Peanut Butter Energy Bites

Preparation Time: 1 hour and 5 minutes

Cooking Time: 0 minute

Servings: 4

Ingredients:

> 1/2 cup oats, old-fashioned
>
> 1/3 cup cocoa powder, unsweetened
>
> 1 cup dates, chopped
>
> 1/2 cup shredded coconut flakes, unsweetened
>
> 1/2 cup peanut butter

Directions:

> Place oats in a food processor along with dates and pulse for 1 minute until the paste starts to come together.
>
> Then add remaining ingredients, and blend until incorporated and very thick mixture comes together.
>
> Shape the mixture into balls, refrigerate for 1 hour until set and then serve.

Nutrition:

Calories: 88.6 Cal

Fat: 5 g

Carbs: 10 g

Protein: 2.3 g

Fiber: 1.6 g

Mango Coconut Cheesecake

Preparation Time: 4 hours and 10 minutes

Cooking Time: 0 minute

Servings: 4

Ingredients:

For the Crust:

> 1 cup macadamia nuts
>
> 1 cup dates, pitted, soaked in hot water for 10 minutes

For the Filling:

> 2 cups cashews, soaked in warm water for 10 minutes
>
> 1/2 cup and 1 tablespoon maple syrup
>
> 1/3 cup and 2 tablespoons coconut oil
>
> 1/4 cup lemon juice
>
> 1/2 cup and 2 tablespoons coconut milk, unsweetened, chilled

For the Topping:

> 1 cup fresh mango slices

Directions:

Prepare the crust, and for this, place nuts in a food processor and process until mixture resembles crumbs.

Drain the dates, add them to the food processor and blend for 2 minutes until thick mixture comes together.

Take a 4-inch cheesecake pan, place date mixture in it, spread and press evenly, and set aside.

Prepare the filling and for this, place all its ingredients in a food processor and blend for 3 minutes until smooth.

Pour the filling into the crust, spread evenly, and then freeze for 4 hours until set.

Top the cake with mango slices and then serve.

Nutrition:

Calories: 200 Cal

Fat: 11 g

Carbs: 22.5 g

Protein: 2 g

Fiber: 1 g

Rainbow Fruit Salad

Preparation Time: 10 minutes

Cooking Time: 0 minute

Servings: 4

Ingredients:

For the Fruit Salad:

> 1 pound strawberries, hulled, sliced
>
> 1 cup kiwis, halved, cubed
>
> 1 1/4 cups blueberries
>
> 1 1/3 cups blackberries
>
> 1 cup pineapple chunks

For the Maple Lime Dressing:

> 2 teaspoons lime zest
>
> 1/4 cup maple syrup
>
> 1 tablespoon lime juice

Directions:

> Prepare the salad, and for this, take a bowl, place all its ingredients and toss until mixed. Prepare the dressing, and for this, take a small bowl, place all its ingredients and whisk well.

Drizzle the dressing over salad, toss until coated and serve.

Nutrition:

Calories: 88.1 Cal

Fat: 0.4 g

Carbs: 22.6 g

Protein: 1.1 g

Fiber: 2.8 g

Cookie Dough Bites

Preparation Time: 4 hours and 10 minutes

Cooking Time: 0 minute

Servings: 18

Ingredients:

- 15 ounces cooked chickpeas
- 1/3 cup vegan chocolate chips
- 1/3 cup and 2 tablespoons peanut butter
- 8 Medjool dates pitted
- 1 teaspoon vanilla extract, unsweetened
- 2 tablespoons maple syrup
- 1 1/2 tablespoons almond milk, unsweetened

Directions:

Place chickpeas in a food processor along with dates, butter, and vanilla and then process for 2 minutes until smooth.

Add remaining ingredients, except for chocolate chips, and then pulse for 1 minute until blends and dough comes together.

Add chocolate chips, stir until just mixed, then shape the mixture into 18 balls and refrigerate for 4 hours until firm.

Serve straight away

Nutrition:

Calories: 200 Cal

Fat: 9 g

Carbs: 26 g

Protein: 1 g

Fiber: 0 g

Dark Chocolate Bars

Preparation Time: 1 hour and 10 minutes

Cooking Time: 2 minutes

Servings: 12

Ingredients:

1 cup cocoa powder, unsweetened

3 Tablespoons cacao nibs

1/8 teaspoon sea salt

2 Tablespoons maple syrup

1 1/4 cup chopped cocoa butter

1/2 teaspoons vanilla extract, unsweetened

2 Tablespoons coconut oil

Directions:

Take a heatproof bowl, add butter, oil, stir, and microwave for 90 to 120 seconds until melts, stirring every 30 seconds.

Sift cocoa powder over melted butter mixture, whisk well until combined, and then stir in maple syrup, vanilla, and salt until mixed.

Distribute the mixture evenly between twelve mini cupcake liners, top with cacao nibs, and freeze for 1 hour until set.

Serve straight away

Nutrition:

Calories: 100 Cal

Fat: 9 g

Carbs: 8 g

Protein: 2 g

Fiber: 2 g

Almond Butter, Oat and Protein Energy Balls

Preparation Time: 1 hour and 10 minutes

Cooking Time: 3 minutes

Servings: 4

Ingredients:

> 1 cup rolled oats
>
> ½ cup honey
>
> 2 ½ scoops of vanilla Protein powder
>
> 1 cup almond butter
>
> Chia seeds for rolling

Directions:

> Take a skillet pan, place it over medium heat, add butter and honey, stir and cook for 2 minutes until warm.
>
> Transfer the mixture into a bowl, stir in Protein powder until mixed, and then stir in oatmeal until combined.
>
> Shape the mixture into balls, roll them into chia seeds, then arrange them on a cookie sheet and refrigerate for 1 hour until firm.

Serve straight away

Nutrition:

Calories: 200 Cal

Fat: 10 g

Carbs: 21 g

Protein: 7 g

Fiber: 4 g

Chocolate and Avocado Truffles

Preparation Time: 1 hour and 10 minutes

Cooking Time: 1 minute

Servings: 18

Ingredients:

> 1 medium avocado, ripe
>
> 2 tablespoons cocoa powder
>
> 10 ounces of dark chocolate chips

Directions:

> Scoop out the flesh from avocado, place it in a bowl, then mash with a fork until smooth, and stir in 1/2 cup chocolate chips.
>
> Place remaining chocolate chips in a heatproof bowl and microwave for 1 minute until chocolate has melted, stirring halfway.
>
> Add melted chocolate into avocado mixture, stir well until blended, and then refrigerate for 1 hour.
>
> Then shape the mixture into balls, 1 tablespoon of mixture per ball, and roll in cocoa powder until covered.
>
> Serve straight away.

Nutrition:

Calories: 59 Cal

Fat: 4 g

Carbs: 7 g

Protein: 0 g

Fiber: 1 g

Coconut Oil Cookies

Preparation Time: 10 minutes

Cooking Time: 10 minutes

Servings: 15

Ingredients:

>   3 1/4 cup oats
>
>   1/2 teaspoons salt
>
>   2 cups coconut Sugar
>
>   1 teaspoons vanilla extract, unsweetened
>
>   1/4 cup cocoa powder
>
>   1/2 cup liquid Coconut Oil
>
>   1/2 cup peanut butter
>
>   1/2 cup cashew milk

Directions:

>   Take a saucepan, place it over medium heat,
>   add all the ingredients except for oats and
>   vanilla, stir until mixed, and then bring the
>   mixture to boil.
>
>   Simmer the mixture for 4 minutes, mixing
>   frequently, then remove the pan from heat
>   and stir in vanilla.

Add oats, stir until well mixed and then scoop
the mixture on a plate lined with wax paper.
Serve straight away.

Nutrition:

Calories: 112 Cal

Fat: 6.5 g

Carbs: 13 g

Protein: 1.4 g

Fiber: 0.1 g

Express Coconut Flax Pudding

Preparation Time: 5 minutes

Cooking Time: 15 minutes

Servings: 4

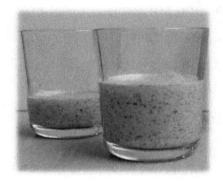

Ingredients:

- 1 Tbsp coconut oil softened
- 1 Tbsp coconut cream
- 2 cups coconut milk canned
- 3/4 cup ground flax seed
- 4 Tbsp coconut palm sugar (or to taste)

Directions:

1. Press SAUTÉ button on your Instant Pot
2. Add coconut oil, coconut cream, coconut milk, and ground flaxseed.
3. Stir about 5 - 10 minutes.

4. Lock lid into place and set on the MANUAL setting for 5 minutes.
5. When the timer beeps, press "Cancel" and carefully flip the Quick Release valve to let the pressure out.
6. Add the palm sugar and stir well.
7. Taste and adjust sugar to taste.
8. Allow pudding to cool down completely.
9. Place the pudding in an airtight container and refrigerate for up to 2 weeks.

Nutrition:

Calories: 140

Fat: 2g

Fiber: 23g

Carbs: 22g

Protein: 47g

Full-flavored Vanilla Ice Cream

Preparation Time: 5 minutes

Cooking Time: 20 minutes

Servings: 8

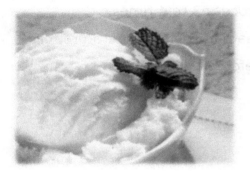

Ingredients:

- 1 1/2 cups canned coconut milk
- 1 cup coconut whipping cream
- 1 frozen banana cut into chunks
- 1 cup vanilla sugar
- 3 Tbsp apple sauce
- 2 tsp pure vanilla extract
- 1 tsp Xanthan gum or agar-agar thickening agent

Directions:

1. Add all ingredients in a food processor; process until all ingredients combined well.

2. Place the ice cream mixture in a freezer-safe container with a lid over.
3. Freeze for at least 4 hours.
4. Remove frozen mixture to a bowl and beat with a mixer to break up the ice crystals.
5. Repeat this process 3 to 4 times.
6. Let the ice cream at room temperature for 15 minutes before serving.

Nutrition:

Calories: 342

Fat: 15g

Fiber: 11g

Carbs: 8g

Protein: 10g

Irresistible Peanut Cookies

Preparation Time: 5 minutes

Cooking Time: 25 minutes

Servings: 8

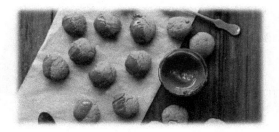

Ingredients:

4 Tbsp all-purpose flour

1 tsp baking soda

pinch of salt

1/3 cup granulated sugar

1/3 cup peanut butter softened

3 Tbsp applesauce

1/2 tsp pure vanilla extract

Directions:

Preheat oven to 350 F.

Combine the flour, baking soda, salt, and sugar in a
mixing bowl; stir.

Add all remaining ingredients and stir well to form a dough.

Roll dough into cookie balls/patties.

Arrange your cookies onto greased (with oil or cooking spray) baking sheet.

Bake for about 8 to 10 minutes.

Let cool for at least 15 minutes before removing from tray.

Remove cookies from the tray and let cool completely.

Place your peanut butter cookies in an airtight container, and keep refrigerated up to 10 days.

Nutrition:

Calories: 211

Fat: 18g

Fiber: 20g

Carbs: 17g

Protein: 39g

Murky Almond Cookies

Preparation Time: 10 minutes

Cooking Time: 15 minutes

Servings: 12

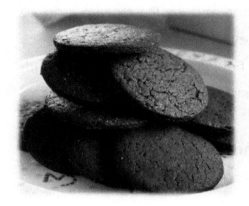

Ingredients:

4 Tbsp cocoa powder

2 cups almond flour

1/4 tsp salt

1/2 tsp baking soda

5 Tbsp coconut oil melted

2 Tbsp almond milk

1 1/2 tsp almond extract

1 tsp vanilla extract

4 Tbsp corn syrup or honey

Directions:

Preheat oven to 340 F degrees.

Grease a large baking sheet; set aside.

Combine the cocoa powder, almond flour, salt, and baking soda in a bowl.

In a separate bowl, whisk melted coconut oil, almond milk, almond and vanilla extract, and corn syrup or honey.

Combine the almond flour mixture with the almond milk mixture and stir until all ingredients incorporate well.

Roll tablespoons of the dough into balls, and arrange onto a prepared baking sheet.

Bake for 12 to 15 minutes.

Remove from the oven and transfer onto a plate lined with a paper towel.

Allow cookies to cool down completely and store in an airtight container at room temperature for about four days.

Nutrition:

Calories: 508

Fat: 12g

Fiber: 9g

Carbs: 24g, Protein: 40g

Orange Semolina Halva

Preparation Time: 15 minutes

Cooking Time: 5 minutes

Servings: 12

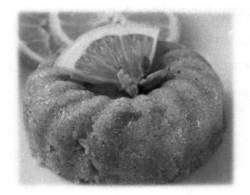

Ingredients:

6 cups fresh orange juice

Zest from 3 oranges

3 cups brown sugar

1 1/4 cup semolina flour

1 Tbsp almond butter (plain, unsalted)

4 Tbsp ground almond

1/4 tsp cinnamon

Directions:

Heat the orange juice, orange zest with brown
 sugar in a pot.

Stir over medium heat until sugar is dissolved.

Add the semolina flour and cook over low heat for 15 minutes; stir occasionally.

Add almond butter, ground almonds, and cinnamon, and stir well.

Cook, frequently stirring, for further 5 minutes.

Transfer the halva mixture into a mold, let it cool and refrigerate for at least 4 hours.

Keep refrigerated in a sealed container for one week.

Nutrition:

Calories: 285

Fat: 28g

Fiber: 7g

Carbs: 34g

Protein: 23g

Seasoned Cinnamon Mango Popsicles

Preparation Time: 15 minutes

Cooking Time: 0 minute

Servings: 6

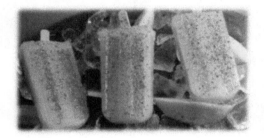

Ingredients:

- 1 1/2 cups of mango pulp
- 1 mango cut in cubes
- 1 cup brown sugar (packed)
- 2 Tbsp lemon juice freshly squeezed
- 1 tsp cinnamon
- 1 pinch of salt

Directions:

Add all ingredients into your blender.

Blend until brown sugar dissolved.

Pour the mango mixture evenly in popsicle molds or
cups.

Insert sticks into each mold.

Place molds in a freezer, and freeze for at least 5 to
6 hours.

Before serving, un-mold easy your popsicles placing
molds under lukewarm water.

Nutrition:

Calories: 423

Fat: 2g

Fiber: 0g

Carbs: 20g

Protein: 33g

Strawberry Molasses Ice Cream

Preparation Time: 20 minutes

Cooking Time: 0 minute

Servings: 8

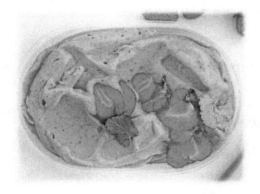

Ingredients:

1 lb strawberries

3/4 cup coconut palm sugar (or granulated sugar)

1 cup coconut cream

1 Tbsp molasses

1 tsp balsamic vinegar

1/2 tsp agar-agar

1/2 tsp pure strawberry extract

Directions:

Add strawberries, date sugar, and the balsamic
vinegar in a blender; blend until completely
combined.

Place the mixture in the refrigerator for one hour.

In a mixing bowl, beat the coconut cream with an
electric mixer to make a thick mixture.

Add molasses, balsamic vinegar, agar-agar, and
beat for further one minute or until combined
well.

Keep frozen in a freezer-safe container (with plastic
film and lid over).

Nutrition:

Calories: 110

Fat: 31g

Fiber: 18g

Carbs: 15g

Protein: 12g

Strawberry-Mint Sorbet

Preparation Time: 10 minutes

Cooking Time: 5 minutes

Servings: 6

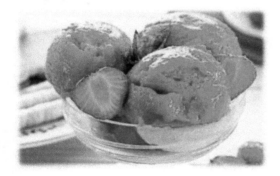

Ingredients:

1 cup of granulated sugar

1 cup of orange juice

1 lb frozen strawberries

1 tsp pure peppermint extract

Directions:

Add sugar and orange juice in a saucepan.

Stir over high heat and boil for 5 minutes or until
sugar dissolves.

Remove from the heat and let it cool down.

Add strawberries into a blender, and blend until
smooth.

Pour syrup into strawberries, add peppermint
extract and stir until all ingredients combined
well.

Transfer mixture to a storage container, cover
tightly, and freeze until ready to serve.

Nutrition:

Calories: 257

Fat: 13g

Fiber: 37g

Carbs: 11g

Protein: 8g

Keto Chocolate Brownies

Preparation Time: 15 minutes

Cooking Time: 15 minutes

Servings: 4

Ingredients:

¼ t. of the following:

salt

baking soda

½ c. of the following:

sweetener of your choice

coconut flour

vegetable oil

water

¼ c. of the following:

cocoa powder

almond milk yogurt

1 tbsp. ground flax

1 t. vanilla extract

Directions:

Bring the oven to 350 heat setting.

Mix the ground flax, vanilla, yogurt, oil, and water;
set to the side for 10 minutes.

Line an oven-safe 8x8 baking dish with parchment paper.

After 10 minutes have passed, add coconut flour, cocoa powder, sweetener, baking soda, and salt.

Bake for 15 minutes; make sure that you placed it in the center. When they come out, they will look underdone.

Place in the refrigerator and let them firm up overnight.

Nutrition:

Calories: 208

Fat: 3g

Fiber: 4g

Carbs: 7g

Protein: 27g

Chocolate Fat Bomb

Preparation Time: 5 minutes

Cooking Time: 0 minutes

Servings: 14

Ingredients:

1 tbsp. liquid sweetener of your choice.

¼ c. of the following:

coconut oil, melted

cocoa powder

½ c. almond butter

Directions:

Mix the ingredients in a medium bowl until smooth.

Pour into the candy molds or ice cube trays.

Put in the freezer to set.

Store in freezer.

Nutrition:

Calories: 241

Fat: 2g

Fiber: 16g

Carbs: 9g

Protein: 22g

Vanilla Cheesecake

Preparation Time: 3 hours 20 minutes

Cooking Time: 0 minute

Servings: 10

Ingredients:

1 tbsp. vanilla extract,

2 ½ tbsp. lemon juice

½ c. coconut oil

1/8 t. stevia powder

6 tbsp. coconut milk

1 ½ c. blanched almonds soaked

Crust:

2 tbsp. coconut oil

1 ½ c. almonds

Directions:

For the Crust:

In a food processor, add the almonds and coconut oil and pulse until crumbles start to form.

Line a 7-inch springform pan with parchment paper and firmly press the crust into the bottom.

For the Sauce:

Bring a saucepan of water to a boil and soak the
almonds for 2 hours. Drain and shake to dry.

Next, add the almonds to the food processor and
blend until completely smooth.

Add vanilla, lemon, coconut oil, stevia, and coconut
milk and blend until smooth.

Pour over the crust and freeze overnight or for a
minimum of 3 hours.

Serve and enjoy.

Nutrition:

Calories: 267

Fat: 13g

Fiber: 14g

Carbs: 17g

Protein: 10g

Chocolate Mousse

Preparation Time: 5 minutes

Cooking Time: 0 minute

Servings: 2

Ingredients:

6 drops liquid stevia extract

½ t. cinnamon

3 tbsp. cocoa powder, unsweetened

1 c. coconut milk

Directions:

On the day before, place the coconut milk into the refrigerator overnight.

Remove the coconut milk from the refrigerator; it should be very thick.

Whisk in cocoa powder with an electric mixer.

Add stevia and cinnamon and whip until combined.

Place in individual bowls and serve and enjoy.

Nutrition:

Calories: 130

Fat: 5g

Fiber: 3g ,Carbs: 6g,Protein: 7g

Peach Sorbet

Preparation time: 15 minutes

Cooking time: 3 hours

Servings: 4

Ingredients:

- 5 Peaches, Peeled, Pitted, And Chopped

- 3/4 Cup Sugar

- Juice of 1 Lemon, or 1 Tablespoon Prepared Lemon Juice

Direction:

1. In the bowl of a food processor, combine all the **Ingredients:** and process until smooth.

2. Pour the mixture into a 9-by-13-inch glass pan. Cover tightly with plastic wrap. Freeze for 3 to 4 hours.

3. Remove from the freezer and scrape the sorbet into a food processor. Process until smooth. Freeze for another 30 minutes, then serve.

Nutrition:

Calories: 291

Fat: 2.3

Fiber: 1.5

Carbs: 34.4

Protein: 5.4

Lime and Watermelon Granita

Preparation time: 15 minutes

Cooking time: 0 minutes

Servings: 4

Ingredients:

- 8 cups seedless -watermelon chunks

- Juice of 2 limes, or 2 tablespoons prepared lime juice

- 1/2 Cup sugar

- Strips of lime zest, for garnish

Directions:

1. In a blender or food processor, combine the watermelon, lime juice, and sugar and process until smooth. You may have to do this in two batches.

2. After processing, stir well to combine both batches.

3. Pour the mixture into a 9-by-13-inch glass dish. Freeze for 2 to 3 hours.

4. Remove from the freezer and use a fork to scrape the top layer of ice. Leave the shaved ice on top and return to the freezer.

5. In another hour, remove from the freezer and repeat. Do this a few more times until all the ice is scraped up. Serve frozen, -garnished with strips of lime zest.

Nutrition:

Calories: 291

Fat: 2.3

Fiber: 1.5

Carbs: 34.4

Protein: 5.4

Chocolate Pudding

Preparation time: 5 minutes

Cooking time: 15 minutes

Servings: 4

Ingredients:

- 1/3 cup sugar

- 1/3 cup unsweetened cocoa powder

- 3 cups unsweetened almond milk

- 1/4 Cup cornstarch

- Pinch of sea salt

- 1 teaspoon vanilla extract

Directions:

1. In a medium bowl, whisk together the sugar and cocoa powder to thoroughly combine.

2. In a large saucepan over medium heat, whisk together the cocoa mixture and 2 1/2 cups of the almond milk.

3. Bring to a boil, stirring constantly. Remove from the heat.

4. In a small bowl, whisk together the remaining 1/2 cup almond milk and cornstarch. Stir into the cocoa mixture and return to medium heat. Add the salt.

5. Stirring constantly, bring the pudding to a boil. It will begin to thicken. Boil for 1 minute. Remove from the heat and stir in the vanilla. Chill before serving.

Nutrition:

Calories: 191

Fat: 2.3

Fiber: 1.5

Carbs: 24.4

Protein: 7.4

Peanut Butter and Crisped Rice Treats

Preparation time: 5 minutes

Cooking time: 5 minutes

Servings: 24

Ingredients:

- 6 cups crisped rice cereal

- 1 cup corn syrup

- 1 cup sugar

- 1 cup chunky peanut butter

Directions:

1. Put the cereal in a large bowl. In a small saucepan, combine the corn syrup and sugar over medium-high heat.

2. Cook, stirring constantly, until the mixture boils. Remove from the heat and stir in the peanut butter. Pour over the cereal and mix to combine.

3. Spread in a 9-by-13-inch pan. Chill for 1
   hour and then cut into squares and serve.

Nutrition:

Calories: 231

Fat: 2.3

Fiber: 2.5

Carbs: 24.4

Protein: 9.4

Caramelized Pears with Balsamic Glaze

Preparation time: 5 minutes

Cooking time: 15 minutes

Servings: 4

Ingredients:

- 1 cup balsamic vinegar

- 1/4 cup plus 3 tablespoons brown sugar

- 1/4 teaspoon grated nutmeg

- Pinch of sea salt

- 1/ cup coconut oil

- 4 pears, cored and cut into slices

Directions:

1. In a medium saucepan, heat the balsamic vinegar, 1/ cup of the brown sugar, the nutmeg, and salt over medium-high heat, stirring to thoroughly incorporate the sugar.

2. Allow to simmer, stirring occasionally, until the glaze reduces by half, 10 to 15 minutes.

3. Meanwhile, heat the coconut oil in a large sauté pan over medium-high heat until it shimmers. Add the pears to the pan in a single layer.

4. Cook until they turn golden, about 5 minutes. Add the remaining 3 tablespoons brown sugar and continue to cook, stirring occasionally, until the pears caramelize, about 5 minutes more.

5. Place the pears on a plate. Drizzle with balsamic glaze and serve.

Nutrition:

Calories: 268

Fat: 2.3

Fiber: 1.5

Carbs: 25.4

Protein: 7.4

Mixed Berries and Cream

Preparation time: 10 minutes

Cooking time: 0 minutes

Servings: 4

Ingredients:

- Two 15-ounce cans full-Fat coconut milk

- 3 tablespoons agave

- 1/2 teaspoon vanilla extract

- 1 pint fresh blueberries

- 1 pint fresh raspberries

- 1 pint fresh strawberries, sliced

Directions:

1. Refrigerate the coconut milk overnight. When you open the can, the liquid will have separated from the solids. Spoon out the solids and reserve the liquid for another purpose.

2. In a medium bowl, whisk the agave and vanilla extract into the coconut solids.

3. Divide the berries among four bowls. Top
   with the coconut cream. Serve immediately.

Nutrition:

Calories: 291

Fat: 2.3

Fiber: 1.5

Carbs: 34.4

Protein: 5.4

Spiced Apple Compote

Preparation time: 15 minutes

Cooking time: 13 minutes

Servings: 4

Ingredients:

- 4 sweet-tart apples, cored and peeled

- 1/2 Cup apple juice

- Juice of 1 lemon

- 1/4 cup brown sugar

- 1/4 teaspoon grated nutmeg

- 1 teaspoon ground cinnamon

- Pinch of Sea Salt

- 1/2 cup chopped pecans

Direction:

1. In a saucepan, cook the apples, apple juice, lemon juice, brown sugar, nutmeg, cinnamon, and salt over medium-high heat, stirring occasionally, until the apples are tender, about 10 minutes.

2. Remove from the heat and set aside.

3. Meanwhile, in a dry sauté pan over medium-high heat, toast the pecans, stirring frequently, about 3 minutes.

4. Serve the compote warm topped with toasted pecans.

Nutrition:

Calories: 198

Fat: 2.3

Fiber: 1.5

Carbs: 19.4

Protein: 4.4

Spiced Rhubarb Sauce

Preparation time: 10 minutes

Cooking time: 15 minutes

Servings: 4

Ingredients:

- 1/2 cup water

- 1/2 cup sugar

- 1/4 teaspoon grated nutmeg

- 1/4 teaspoon ground ginger

- 1/4 teaspoon ground cinnamon

- 1 pound rhubarb, cut into 1/2- to 1-inch pieces

Directions:

1. In a large saucepan, bring the water, sugar, nutmeg, ginger, and cinnamon to a boil.

2. Add the rhubarb and cook over medium-high heat, stirring frequently, until the -rhubarb is soft and saucy, about 10 minutes.

3. Chill for at least 30 minutes before -serving.

Nutrition:

Calories: 261

Fat: 2.3

Fiber: 1.5

Carbs: 14.4

Protein: 10.4

Coconut and Almond Truffles

Preparation time: 15 minutes

Cooking time: 0 minutes

Servings: 8

Ingredients:

- 1 cup pitted dates

- 1 cup almonds

- 1/2 cup sweetened cocoa powder, plus extra for coating

- 1/2 cup unsweetened shredded coconut

- 1/4 cup pure maple syrup

- 1 teaspoon vanilla extract

- 1 teaspoon almond extract

- 1/4 Teaspoon sea salt

Directions:

1. In the bowl of a food processor, combine all the **Ingredients:** and process until smooth. Chill the mixture for about 1 hour.

2. Roll the mixture into balls and then roll the balls in cocoa powder to coat. Serve immediately or keep chilled until ready to serve.

Nutrition:

Calories: 234

Fat: 2.3

Fiber: 1.5

Carbs: 20.4

Protein: 6.4

Chocolate Macaroons

Preparation time: 10 minutes

Cooking time: 15 minutes

Servings: 8

Ingredients:

- 1 cup unsweetened shredded coconut

- 2 tablespoons cocoa powder

- 2/3 cup coconut milk

- 1/4 cup agave

- Pinch of sea salt

Directions:

1. Preheat the oven to 350 degree F. Line a baking sheet with parchment paper.

2. In a medium saucepan, cook all the **Ingredients:** over -medium-high heat until a firm dough is formed.

3. Scoop the dough into balls and place on the baking sheet. Bake for 15 minutes, remove

from the oven, and let cool on the baking
sheet.

4. Serve cooled macaroons or store in a tightly
   sealed container for up to 1 week.

Nutrition:

Calories: 291

Fat: 2.3

Fiber: 1.5

Carbs: 34.4

Protein: 5.4

Tangy Heirloom Carrot

Preparation Time: 10 minutes

Cooking Time: 45 minutes

Serving: 6

Ingredients

    1 bunch heirloom carrots

    1 tablespoon fresh thyme leaves

    ½ tablespoon coconut oil

    1 tablespoon date paste

    1/8 cup freshly-squeezed orange juice

    1/8 teaspoon salt

    Extra salt if needed

Direction

    1.   Preheat your oven to 350 degrees Fahrenheit

    2.   Wash carrots and discard green pieces

    3.   Take a small-sized bowl and add coconut oil, orange juice, salt, and date paste

    4.   Pour mixture over carrots and spread on a large baking sheet

5.   Sprinkle thyme and roast for 45 minutes

6.   Sprinkle salt on top and enjoy!

Nutrition

106 Calories

2g Fat

2g Protein

Just Apple Slices

Preparation Time: 10 minutes

Cooking Time: 10 minutes

Serving: 4

Ingredients

    1 cup of coconut oil

    ¼ cup date paste

    2 tablespoons ground cinnamon

    4 granny smith apples, peeled and sliced, cored

Direction

    1.   Take a large-sized skillet and place it over medium heat

    2.   Add oil and allow the oil to heat up

    3.   Stir in cinnamon and date paste into the oil

    4.   Add cut up apples and cook for 5-8 minutes until crispy

    5.   Serve and enjoy!

Nutrition

368 Calories

23g Fat, 1g Protein

Vegan Mini Gingerbread Loaves

Preparation Time: 15 minutes

Cooking Time: 30 minutes

Servings: 8

Ingredients:

For Gingerbread

- 3 cups gluten-free flour

- 2 teaspoons baking powder

- teaspoon baking soda

- 1 1/2 teaspoons cinnamon

- 1 1/2 teaspoons ground ginger

- 1 cup coconut milk, unsweetened

- 1 cup coconut sugar

- ½ cup unsweetened applesauce

- ½ cup pumpkin puree

- 2/3 cup canola oil

- ½ cup molasses

- 1 teaspoon vanilla extract

For the Ginger Vanilla Glaze

- 1/2 cup powdered sugar

- tablespoon coconut milk

- ½ teaspoon ground ginger

- ½ teaspoon pure vanilla extract

Directions:

For Gingerbread

1. Preheat oven to 350ºF.

2. Spray small loaf pans with cooking spray or line with parchment paper.

3. Sift together flour, baking powder, soda, cinnamon, salt, and ginger. Mix well.

4. Mix coconut milk, applesauce, pumpkin puree, vanilla, oil, and molasses.

5. Add liquid ingredients to the dry mixture, and stir to combine.

6. Pour batter into the small loaf pans.

7. Bake for 30 minutes until a toothpick inserted into the center of the gingerbread comes out clean.

8. Cool desserts for 10 minutes before removing from pan.

For Glaze

1. Mix powdered sugar, coconut milk, vanilla, and ginger in a blender.

2. Drizzle glaze over cooled gingerbread.

Nutrition:

Calories: 579

Fat: 26g

Carbs: 99g

Sugar: 24g

Protein: 5g

Vegan Chocolate Turron

Preparation Time: 10 minutes

Cooking Time: 5 minutes

Servings: 16

Ingredients:

- ½ lb. dark chopped chocolate

- 2 tablespoons melted coconut oil

- 2 oz. unsalted raw hazelnuts

Directions:

1. Place dark chocolate in a saucepan. Cook over medium heat, stirring occasionally until chocolate is melted.

2. Remove chocolate from the heat. Add hazelnuts, and combine well.

3. Pour the chocolate-hazelnuts mixture into lined rectangular dish.

4. Cool to room temperature. Chop the Turron.

5. If it's too hot in the room, keep Turron in the fridge.

Nutrition:

Calories: 120

Protein: 2g

Fat: 10g

Sugar 8g

Carbs: 10g

Vegan Chocolate Orange Truffles

Preparation Time: 15 minutes

Cooking Time: 0 minute

Servings: 16

Ingredients:

- ½ lb. pitted dates

- 2 oz. almond meal

- 2 tablespoons unsweetened cocoa powder

- 2 teaspoons cocoa powder (for rolling the balls)

- 2 tablespoons orange juice

- lemon peel

Directions:

1. Place pitted dates, almond meal, cocoa powder, orange juice, and lemon zest in a food processor or a powerful blender. Mix well.

2. Make the mixture into balls using your hands. Make 16 truffles.

3. Roll the candies in cocoa powder to taste.

Nutrition:

Calories: 58

Protein: 1g

Fat: 2g

Sugar 3g

Carbs: 11g

Gluten-Free Chocolate Orange Vegan Cake

Preparation Time: 10 minutes

Cooking Time: 40 minute

Servings: 8

Ingredients:

For the Cake

- 3 tablespoons flax seeds

- 6 tablespoons water

- 4 oz. gluten-free oat flour

- 2 oz. unsweetened cocoa powder

- 4 oz. brown sugar

- teaspoon baking soda

- 1 teaspoon baking powder

- ½ cup agave syrup

- 1 cup orange juice

- tablespoons extra virgin olive oil

- 1 tablespoon orange marmalade

For Chocolate Frosting

- 125 ml water

- ½ lb. dates

- 2 tablespoons unsweetened cocoa powder

- 4 tablespoons orange juice

- tablespoon orange marmalade

Directions:

For the Cake

1. Preheat the oven to 355ºF.

2. Place flax seeds and water in a blender. Blend well.

3. Mix chickpea flour, cocoa powder, sugar, oat flour, baking powder, and soda in a bowl.

4. Mix blended flax seeds, agave syrup, orange juice, marmalade, and oil in another bowl.

5. Mix wet and dry ingredients until smooth.

6. Put parchment paper on a bottom of the sheet Pour the mixture into a deep baking dish. Bake for 40 minutes.

For the Frosting

1. Mix all the ingredients with a blender until smooth.

2. Spread the mixture over the cooled cake.

Nutrition:

Calories: 200

Protein: 3g

Fat 4g

Sugar 5g

Carbs: 40g

Coconut Snowballs

Preparation Time: 20 minutes, 1 week for freezing

Cooking Time: 0 minute

Servings: 10

Ingredients:

- 3 oz. shredded coconut

- 1-oz. almond flour

- 3 oz. agave syrup

Directions:

1. Mix shredded coconut, flour, and syrup in a food processor until well combined.

2. Make 10 balls using your hands.

3. Roll the balls in 1 oz. shredded coconut.

4. You can keep these balls in a sealed container in a fridge for one week.

Nutrition:

Calories: 88,Protein: 1g,Fat 5g,Sugar: 4g

Carbs: 9g

Champagne Jelly with Fruits and Berries

Preparation Time: 20 minutes

Cooking Time: 0 minute

Servings: 4

Ingredients:

- 500 ml semi-sweet champagne

- 1/3-oz. agar-agar powder

- medium pear

- 1 medium peach

- 1 medium nectarine

- 2-3 apricots

- 5 oz. seedless grapes

- 5 oz. sweet cherries

- 5 oz. strawberries

Directions:

1. Wash fruits and berries well.

2. Peel the fruits and berries. Cut into pieces. Leave the grapes and other small berries for decorating.

3. Pour agar-agar into the champagne in a deep saucepan and place on low heat. Stir until the gelatin dissolves. Remove from heat.

4. Line the jelly containers with plastic wrap.

5. Place the fruits and berries in a container. Pour champagne over fruit.

6. Refrigerate for 5-6 hours. Turn the container over and remove the plastic wrap.

Nutrition:

Calories: 134

Protein: 2g

Fat 1g

Sugar 5g

Carbs: 32

Oranges with Cinnamon and Honey

Preparation Time: 5 minutes

Cooking Time: 15 minute

Servings: 4 servings

Ingredients:

- 10 1/2 oz. orange
- 4 tablespoons honey
- teaspoon cinnamon
- 1 oz. walnuts

Directions:

1. Peel the oranges, divide into slices.

2. Place the slices on a baking dish.

3. Chop the nuts.

4. Mix honey with cinnamon and nuts.

5. Sprinkle honey-nut mixture on oranges slices.

6. Preheat the oven to 390 ºF. Then place the baking sheet in the oven and bake for 15 minutes.

7. You can eat orange slices cool or warm.

Nutrition:

Calories: 179

Protein: 2g

Fat: 5g

Sugar: 5g

Carbs: 32g

Green Buckwheat Coffee Cake

Preparation Time: 20 minutes

Cooking Time: 30 minutes

Servings: 8

Ingredients:

For the Cake Base

- 15 bright dates

- 2 tablespoons cocoa

- cup walnuts (or other to your taste)

For the Filling

- 1/8 cup green buckwheat

- cup plain milk

- 15 dates

- teaspoons chicory

- teaspoons cocoa

- ½-1 cup milk (additional)

Directions:

For the Base

1. Soak dates overnight to soften. Remove the pits from the dates and blend them in a food processor.

2. Peel the walnuts, and grind nuts into crumbs.

3. Add cocoa to the nuts.

4. Mix half the dates, nuts and cocoa with a fork until smooth. Make into balls with wet hands. If the dough is too thin, add cocoa or nuts.

5. Spread the dough on the bottom of a medium middle baking sheet.

For the Filling

1. Grind the green buckwheat into flour using a coffee grinder.

2. Place the buckwheat flour in a saucepan. Add a little milk and stir well until no lumps remain.

3. Warm up the mixture and boil until it thickens (for 5-10 minutes).

4. Place the second half of the dates, chicory, cocoa and a little milk in a food processor. Beat into thick, homogeneous cream. Add milk as needed.

5. Place the mixture on top of the base. Freeze cake for 2-3 hours. If the cake is too frozen, let it stand at room temperature for 15-20 minutes.

6. Coat the cake with the melted chocolate or icing.

Nutrition:

Calories: 328

Protein: 8g

Fat: 19g

Sugar: 10g

Carbs: 33g

Sweet Chocolate Hummus

Preparation Time: 10 minutes

Cooking Time: 5 minutes

Servings: 3

Ingredients:

- 2 tablespoons boiled chickpeas

- 4 full tablespoons cocoa

- 4 tablespoons honey

- tablespoon orange juice

- 5 tablespoons oil, coconut or peanut

- 1/5 teaspoon cinnamon, nutmeg or vanilla (optional)

Directions:

1. Boil the chickpeas. After cooking rinse and drain excess liquid.

2. Put chickpeas, honey, cocoa, softened butter and spices in a blender bowl. Pour in 2/3 cups of milk. If necessary, mix by hand, folding from the bottom up.

3. If it is hard for the blender to mix, add a little milk to get a smooth chocolate mixture without grains.

4. If hummus is not sweet enough, add honey or syrup.

Nutrition:

Calories: 432

Protein: 7g

Fat: 29g

Sugar: 10g

Carbs: 35g

Fruits and Berries in Orange Juice Salad

Preparation Time: 10 minutes

Cooking Time: 0 minute

Servings: 2

Ingredients:

- cup strawberries

- 1 cup sweet cherries

- 1/2 cup of blueberries

- 1 red apple

- 1 peach

- 1 kiwi

- 1 cup of orange juice

- tablespoons lemon juice

Directions:

1. Wash and halve the cherries. Remove the pits. Put cherries on a deep plate.

2. Then, wash and cut strawberries into quarters. Add strawberries to the cherries.

3. Add washed blueberries.

4. Wash, cut, and peel the apple, peach, and kiwi. Add the pieces to the other ingredients.

5. Mix all fruits and berries. Pour orange juice over fruit mixture.

6. Add two tablespoons of lemon juice. Let the salad soak up the citrus, and then drain the juice. Eat chilled.

Nutrition:

Calories: 342

Protein: 3g

Fat: 1g

Carbs: 52g

Tropical Fruits Salad

Preparation Time: 10 minutes

Cooking Time: 0 minute

Servings: 2

Ingredients:

- pineapple

- mangoes

- bananas

- 1/2 cup pomegranate seeds

- 2 tablespoons sweet coconut shavings

Directions:

1. Wash, peel and cut pineapple, mango and bananas into medium cubes. Put fruits in a deep plate.

2. Add the pomegranate seeds to the dish, mix and let stand for several hours in the refrigerator.

3. Sprinkle with coconut flakes before eating.

Nutrition:

Calories: 297

Protein: 5g

Fat: 6g

Sugar: 8g

Carbs: 10g

Paste (Halva)

Preparation Time: 10 minutes

Cooking Time: 0 minute

Servings: 10

Ingredients:

- 7 oz. peanuts

- 40 ml sunflower oil

- 1/3 cup sugar

- 70 ml water

- 1/3 cup wheat flour

- teaspoon vanilla sugar

Directions:

1. Peel the peanuts. Fry in a clean and dry pan for 3-5 minutes, stirring constantly.

2. Pour the wheat flour into another pan, stirring with a spoon. Fry until creamy.

3. Remove from the heat.

4. Grind the peanuts in food processers as finely as possible.

5. Pour the fried flour in the food processor. Grind for 2 minutes.

6. Place sugar, vanilla sugar and water in a small saucepan. Bring to a boil. Boil the syrup for one minute. Add vegetable oil, mix the ingredients, and remove from heat.

7. Pour the syrup into the peanut mixture. Mix well. The mass thickens quite quickly.

8. Put the mass into the mold. Line the form with parchment paper for easy removal. Leave the halva to cool completely.

9. The paste is ready. Cut into pieces and try!

10. Halva can be from golden to brown, depending on the degree the flour and peanuts are roasted.

Nutrition:

Calories: 197

Protein: 6g

Fat: 13g

Sugar: 11g

Carbs: 11g

Peanut Butter Quinoa Cups

Preparation Time: 10 minutes

Cooking Time: 0 minute

Servings: 6

Ingredients:

- 4oz. puffed quinoa

- 2oz. smooth peanut butter

- 1.5oz. coconut butter

- 30ml coconut oil

- 25ml maple syrup

- 5ml vanilla extract

Directions:

1. Combine peanut butter, coconut butter, and coconut oil in a microwave-safe bowl.

2. Microwave on high until melted, in 40-second intervals.

3. Stir in the puffed quinoa. Stir gently to combine.

4. Divide the mixture among 12 paper cases.

    Freeze for 1 hour

Nutrition:

Calories: 231

Carbs: 12g

Fat: 9g

Protein: 6.3g

Conclusion

In a nutshell, this cookbook offers you a world full of options to diversify your plant-based menu. People on this diet are usually seen struggling to choose between healthy food and flavor but, soon, they run out of the options. The selection of 250 recipes in this book is enough to adorn your dinner table with flavorsome, plant-based meals every day. Give each recipe a good read and try them out in the kitchen. You will experience tempting aromas and binding flavors every day.

The book is conceptualized with the idea of offering you a comprehensive view of a plant-based diet and how it can benefit the body. You may find the shift sudden, especially if you are a die-hard fan of non-vegetarian items. But you need not give up anything that you love. Eat everything in moderation.

The next step is to start experimenting with the different recipes in this book and see which ones are your favorites. Everyone has their favorite food, and you will surely find several of yours in this book. Start with breakfast and work your way through. You will be pleasantly surprised at how tasty a vegan meal really can be.

You will love reading this book, as it helps you to understand how revolutionary a plant-based diet can be. It will help you to make informed decisions as you move toward greater change for the greater good. What are you waiting for? Have you begun your journey on the path of the plant-based diet yet? If you haven't, do it now! Now you have everything you need to get started making budget-friendly, healthy plant-based recipes. Just follow your basic shopping list and follow your meal plan to get started! It's easy to switch over to a plant-based diet if you have your meals planned out and temptation locked away. Don't forget to clean out your kitchen before starting, and you're sure to meet all your diet and health goals.

You need to plan if you are thinking about dieting. First, you can start slowly by just eating one meal a day, which is vegetarian and gradually increasing your number of vegetarian meals. Whenever you are struggling, ask your friend or family member to support you and keep you motivated. One important thing is also to be regularly accountable for not following the diet.

If dieting seems very important to you and you need to do it right, then it is recommended that you visit a professional such as a nutritionist or dietitian to discuss your dieting plan and optimizing it for the better.

No matter how much you want to lose weight, it is not advised that you decrease your calorie intake to an unhealthy level. Losing weight does not mean that you stop eating. It is done by carefully planning meals.

A plant-based diet is very easy once you get into it. At first, you will start to face a lot of difficulties, but if you start slowly, then you can face all the barriers and achieve your goal.

Swap out one unhealthy food item each week that you know is not helping you and put in its place one of the plant-based ingredients that you like. Then have some fun creating the many different recipes in this book. Find out what recipes you like the most so you can make them often and most of all; have some fun exploring all your recipe options.

Wish you good luck with the plant-based diet!

CPSIA information can be obtained
at www.ICGtesting.com
Printed in the USA
BVHW050836120421
604731BV00002B/106

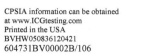

9 781801 833424